Healthy Body, Healthy Brain

Healthy Body, Healthy Brain

Alzheimer's and Dementia Prevention and Care

Jenny Lewis

Floris Books

1/11

I dedicate this book to all who truly *care*
and have the vision to pioneer change.

First published in 2010 by Floris Books

British Library CIP Data available

ISBN 978-086315-750-9

Printed in Poland

As a society we will be judged by future generations on how we care for the very young, the disabled, the sick and the elderly.

We hear, but we do not listen; we listen, but we do not hear.

Contents

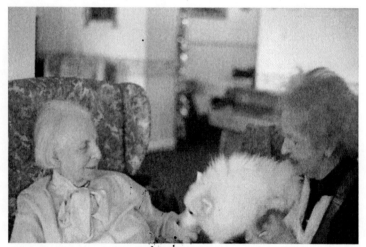

Ruby delights in a visit from Millie, Mary's 'pat dog'.

Introduction

This book is the result of fifteen years of research and experience as a carer for my mother, Ruby, who has suffered from senile dementia for that time. For nine years Ruby was a resident of an EMI (Elderly Mentally Impaired) care home near where we live in Devon. Now, at the age of ninety-three years, my mother is in the final stages of her condition and requires nursing care. I have known despair, anger, frustration, physical and emotional exhaustion and shed many tears. Yet always beneath the layers of seeming helplessness, to prevent a deterioration in my mother's condition, I have fostered hope — hope that there is a way to improve life, both now and throughout the duration of her condition, which in some small measure has been achieved.

I know that my mother, Ruby, who has always shown compassion, great courage and determination throughout her life, would wish me to share my research and experience, to benefit others and to bring hope and raise awareness that there can be a future for people suffering from Alzheimer's and dementia. The old adage holds true: 'If only I knew then what I know now.'

The path has been long and hard, but worth the journey if at least some of the suggestions in this book can be perceived as beneficial and acted upon by those who care for the elderly. If, as a society of individuals, we cared enough for the vulnerable elderly, we would implement essential specialist dementia training programmes for nurses, doctors, care staff and families as a priority! If the will is there, it can be done. The importance of encouraging mobility, and therefore independence, for as long as possible cannot be overstated. Care programmes that offer physiotherapy, daily music and movement help motivate older people — who could otherwise be sitting in a chair for long periods — to use their limbs, and they promote a feeling of well-being.

This is predominantly a practical book, containing what I trust will be seen as helpful suggestions for present and future carers who want to find the best and simplest ways to help those in their care to attain a healthy and fulfilled older age. There is special emphasis on the prevention of Alzheimer's and dementia as well as suggestions on how to improve the health and well-being of those who already have these conditions.

1. Challenges that face us as we grow older

The challenge of ageing well is one of the greatest issues facing society in this country today. Predicted demographic changes show us that life expectancy is set to increase by two years per decade. This means that many of us living now can expect to gain about six minutes of life every half an hour!

At the present time, there are 750,000 people in this country with dementia, with the figures set to rise to 900,000 in five years time and to just under two million by 2050.

In the British Isles we have more than 10,000 people over the age of 100 years, and it is estimated that by 2020 or sooner this figure will rise to 90,000. How are we going to add purpose to life and see these years as a gift, rather than as years to be endured with debilitating physical and mental deterioration?

Researchers have found that keeping a positive outlook, instead of descending into negativity, fatalism and denial about the process of ageing, becomes a key factor in maintaining enjoyment at any age, especially as we grow older. The more effort that we put into understanding the physical and mental processes of ageing, the more we will discover how we can age well and go on to live fulfilled lives, even into our nineties and 100s. People do!

I am sure we were all moved by the words and dedication of Henry Allingham, the 109 year-old and last survivor of the

Battle of Jutland. Henry travelled to France in 2005 to lay a wreath at the memorial service to honour those who fought in the First World War. Henry was fit enough to make the journey, and he was mentally alert.

In 2007 Henry's golf club held a dinner in honour of his 111th birthday. Among the reasons given for his long life, Henry told of how he'd always cycled and only gave up when he was 100 years old. He'd also always been an active golfer.

2. Strengths and weaknesses that help or hinder

It is obvious that bad health, illness and disability can seriously erode our quality of life. However, even in these circumstances, a positive attitude can assist the healing process and help to make each day happier. Put simply, a proverbial cup can be half full or half empty. The earlier in life that we recognize the possible consequences of a negative attitude, the sooner we can prepare a healthy attitude for our later years.

Of course, if we live in a care situation, that is, either receiving care in our own home or in a residential or nursing home, then the people who care for us will need to adopt a similar positive attitude. Here are some basic examples to illustrate what I mean:

Happy Old Age	Miserable Old Age
Positive outlook	Pessimistic outlook
Healthy independence	Unhealthy or reluctant dependence
Control over making decisions	Loss of control; others making decisions
Useful, structured role in life	No obvious role or purpose in life

Happy Old Age	Miserable Old Age
Confidence that life continues to have a purpose	Lack of reason to live
Mentally active and interested in learning	Mentally passive; too much TV; no imaginative stimulation
Physically active	Sedentary; little or no exercise
Socially interactive	Socially isolated and inactive
Good nutrition that improves biology of life	Poor nutrition that starves life force and weakens immune system

Negative states of mind can create stressful situations. Excessive stress ages a person more progressively, both physically and mentally, than someone who has a positive outlook, especially when confronted with making difficult decisions in life.

3. The role of genetic make-up

Although it's true that genetic inheritance plays a role in life, researchers believe that there are no deterministic genes for ageing. Recent research has found that the risk of inheriting Alzheimer's disease is small (Holford, *The Alzheimer's Prevention Plan*, 31). Consequently, gerontologists have discovered that — because we are not wholly genetically programmed — nutrition, lifestyle and a positive or negative attitude play a significant role in whether or not we age well and live a long life. To quote from the June 2007 edition of the Alzheimer's Society magazine, 'Living with Dementia':

> Many people worry they may be at risk of developing dementia if a close relative has the disease. The vast majority of cases of dementia are not inherited, nor are they caused by a genetic fault. Where there is a family link, the disease is referred to as familial Alzheimer's disease and usually affects younger people (under sixty-five) rather than older people, but most cases of early onset dementia are not inherited.

For further information on this subject I'd recommend reading chapter four of *The Alzheimer's Prevention Plan* by Patrick Holford (see *References and resources* for further details).

Dr Otto Wolff describes the process very clearly in his book, *Anthroposophical Medicine and its Remedies* quoted in the *Journal of Anthroposophic Medicine* 1994:

The symptoms of Alzheimer's disease closely resemble those of senile dementia, or cerebral sclerosis, but it would be fair to say that with Alzheimer's disease we evidently have a degenerative process, whilst some degree of senile atrophy is physiologic for all organs. In old age, performance capacity of muscle decreases, as does the elasticity of the lens and acuity of hearing; in principle the function of all organs are reduced. This is necessary, as the used up body will have to be put aside in the end.

However, Dr Wolff continues in a positive vein with the assurance that, as *inactivity* weakens us in body, soul and spirit, so *activity* strengthens and maintains organ function. Physical training will strengthen muscle function, and the brain can likewise be trained and strengthened through mental activity, rather than passively taking in information through TV, advertising and a flood of unconnected stimuli.

It is generally accepted that some memory loss is an inevitable part of growing older. Dr Wolff observed that, although short-term memory is affected, long-term memory is generally remarkably well preserved. Further, he points out that the forgetfulness of old age relates mainly to knowledge of detail, but that it is possible to learn new content. He suggests that in the past, people intuitively knew and understood the wisdom of old age.

4. How to avoid ageism

Ageism, as we often experience it today, trundles along tired paths of limited and outmoded thinking, with attitudes that have been deeply embedded in the ideology of Western society for years. We can all play our part in changing that pattern. There is some evidence that changes are taking place. In his book, *The Importance of Living,* the Chinese scholar Lin Ytang wrote:

In my efforts to compare and contrast Eastern and Western life I have found no differences that are absolute, except one, in the matter of our attitude towards getting older; the difference is absolute and the East and the West take exactly opposite points of view … In China the first question one person asks of another after his name is, 'What is your age?' If the person replies apologetically that he is twenty-three, the other party will comfort him by expressing the hope that one day he may become old. A person who is able to celebrate his eighty-first birthday is looked upon as one specially blessed by heaven and receives honour both from family and community.

As a society we need to change any negative language or attitudes that see older folk as an economic or social burden. For future generations this could be achieved through education by encouraging young people to take an interest in older people, and to experience positive interaction in which they can benefit from the knowledge and experience of older people. In that way, young people can learn to respect and understand the ideas and needs of older people in the twenty-first century. Such interaction would be mutually beneficial.

Older people represent a living source of important first-hand social history, taking into account their subjective as well as their objective experiences. Younger people can offer new and fresh perspectives that keep older people in touch with new thinking and ideas, which can lead to stimulating and lively debates. Schools and colleges should be awake to the possibilities such debates offer! The drive and enthusiasm for change that is part of healthy, growing young people, with the many issues that confront them, can be developed and debated in conversation with older people, who have already experienced the consequences that can result from present-day actions. Whether environmental, political, economic, educational, historical or personal issues, all could benefit from a sharing of views.

An obvious and yet positive truth as we reach our seventies and eighties is that we are forced into making the present count as quality time, given that our future is shortening and plans become increasingly fragile as we move forward.

Ageing is something we all do with the passage of time, but it need not be synonymous with crippling physical or mental degeneration. There are numerous cases of people who it is said 'die healthy' from what could be simply described as 'wear and tear!' How wonderful if, as individuals, we could use past valuable years of experience and learning to make our later years a time of fulfilment and regeneration.

Let us, then, celebrate the growing numbers of elders in our midst as inspiring an important and potentially creative gathering time for us all, as we ourselves prepare to reach that later stage in life. After all, most of us will one day become old and hope that we will be healthy and independent as we age, and continue to be listened to and treated with dignity and respect.

5. A better understanding of Alzheimer's and dementia

From my own fifteen years of experience, and research drawn from many eminent sources, it is clear that most forms of dementia originate from a physical and not a mental cause. This approach is backed up by worldwide research, including that of Dr Rudolf Steiner, the founder of anthroposophical medicine, and the nutritionist, Patrick Holford, whose work is seminal on this subject. Both deserve serious attention. Throughout two of his books, *New Optimum Nutrition for the Mind* and *The Alzheimer's Prevention Plan,* Patrick Holford makes a strong case that both Alzheimer's and senile dementia can be prevented in most cases, and that sufferers will benefit greatly if their condition is treated as a physical illness. As seen with Alzheimer's and senile dementia, a physical illness can affect the mind and not just the body, for example, the ability to think or reason. Mood and decision-making can also be affected and depression is very common, especially as memory progressively declines.

To give a simple example, many of us have experienced influenza or other diseases that cause a high temperature, and have suffered the subsequent light-headed feeling and confusion that affects the mind and distorts perception. Thankfully, the experience is only temporary and passes. With Alzheimer's and many other forms of dementia the confusion does not go away and often worsens over time.

For more information on Alzheimer's disease and the most common causes of dementia, see The Alzheimer's Society website, www.alzheimers.org.uk.

With the help and research of bodies such as the Alzheimer's Society, we are gaining in understanding about Alzheimer's and dementia, and how to treat people with these conditions, especially since people are developing them at an increasingly young age. However, it will take a long time to remove prejudices and negative attitudes from our society and we need to develop more understanding of the causes — prevention being better than cure. The condition must not be relegated to the type of 'asylum' attitude that was so prevalent in past centuries, where people were stigmatized, shut away and forgotten.

In Dorothy Wordsworth's time the condition was called 'faculty-crazed.' Dorothy suffered from it in her latter days and William, along with his wife Mary, looked after her until his death in 1850. Dorothy died five years later. It is interesting that, apparently, William was the only one who could calm Dorothy in her more disturbed moments. This was no doubt due to a lifelong, deep, loving brother and sister friendship, and many years of sharing the same home and literary interests, as well as walking vast distances together over the hills of their beloved Lakeland.

6. How to achieve a miracle — identifying causes and deficiencies

In the twenty-first century, where we have access to worldwide medical expertise, we need to explore and research a variety of avenues in order to better understand and treat this condition. First of all I will outline possible causes and areas of deficiency before moving into areas of supplementation.

It is estimated that around fifty per cent of all problems associated with people suffering from Alzheimer's or age-associated memory disorders are related to:

Depression / stress
Minor strokes to the brain
Long-term alcoholism
Brain injuries
Toxic reaction to drugs
Chronic constipation
Nutritional deficiencies
Heavy-metal excesses in the blood

Nutrition

The digestive tracts of most very elderly people are poor in assimilation and, as a consequence, insufficient nutrients reach cells because of a sluggish digestive system. This is one reason why, in the UK today, it is estimated that over fifty per cent of older people are malnourished: a shocking statistic, and cause for concerted action.

Absorption of nutrients is made worse by constipation that results in the re-absorption of toxins. Drinking plenty of water will help relieve constipation. The condition is exacerbated by loss of mobility, when elderly people don't or are unable to take sufficient exercise, which, as already stated, is often the case in residential homes. A good, well-run and supervised residential or nursing home will make every effort to encourage each individual's mobility.

Blood sugar levels are also critical for the efficient function of the brain, as the sugars in the blood act as the brain's fuel. Low blood sugar levels disrupt concentration and can bio-chemically prevent the brain from storing new memories.

Many of the people who are most prone to memory loss and concentration because of chronic stress are also prone to dietary deficiencies, for the simple reason that stress increases nutritional needs as well as creating over production of cortisol, which I will go on to discuss below in further detail.

Toxins

In an integrated approach, each individual, upon recognising the symptoms of Alzheimer's or dementia and contacting their general practitioner, would benefit from vitamin, mineral and allergy tests to ascertain any toxins or imbalances in the system. It is possible to have tests carried out privately, and laboratories that offer this service are listed under *References and resources*. These procedures are most important in the early stages of these conditions, to identify problems and allow treatment to take place.

Aluminium, although not a heavy metal and naturally present in nature, is now commonly used in foods and in medicines such as antacids, as well as in cosmetics. Some studies have found an excess of aluminium toxicity in the brains of people with Alzheimer's disease. The jury is still out regarding aluminium as a cause of Alztheimer's, but it is probably best to err on the side of caution here. Lead is a neurotoxin and can cause abnormal brain and nerve function. Mercury can cause brain damage. Both are heavy metals, toxic and best avoided. Tests will ascertain whether or not toxins are present, or whether a deficiency or excess in one or more amino acid could be causing the problem. In such cases, treatment can begin to restore full health. In certain cases it would also be appropriate to test for a possible virus.

The research of Peter Bennett, who worked as Chief Constable in the North Yorkshire Police Constabulary, revealed that many young offenders suffered from nutritional deficiencies or stored heavy-metal excesses in the body. He concluded that many ill-health and behavioural symptoms are linked to mineral deficiencies or imbalances, and from storing toxic metals in the body. A successful programme was devised, using tests to determine deficiencies or toxins and then implementing a nutritional diet and supplementation. A similar approach can be used to restore health, or at the very least to bring quality of life, to people suffering from Alzheimer's and dementia.

Excess dietary fat

Vascular plaque, caused by excessive dietary fat, decreases blood flow to the brain cells. *This is critical.* The brain depends upon approximately twenty-five per cent of all blood pumped to the heart, and reduced cerebral circulation has a profoundly negative effect upon the brain. High blood pressure, often caused by poor diet and stress, draws blood away from where it is needed by the brain, thus affecting memory and concentration.

Excess dietary fat produces free radicals that cause millions of neurons to die. The brain needs a constant supply of oxygen and glucose, which is supplied by the blood. If the blood supply is cut off, even for a couple of minutes, then the brain cells in that area will be killed. This happens in vascular dementia, known as multi-infarct — a minor stroke to the brain.

Neurotransmitter deficiency

A nerve cell or neuron is like a radio receiver in that it carries information rapidly from one part of the brain to another. But there is a tiny gap called a synapse between each neuron and its neighbour in its circuitry. We, the listeners, hear the message because a chemical messenger, a neurotransmitter, leaps across the gap and passes on the message. What neurotransmitters need to build up these messages are amino acids, which are taken into the body through the food we eat. To complete our analogy of the radio receiver, deficiencies of amino acids mean a break in transmission and therefore the message does not get through; in terms of our brain, the 'hardware' of the mind can no longer carry our thoughts.

There are some forty amino acids, and the subject is clearly expanded by Patrick Holford in chapter five of his book, *The Alzheimer's Prevention Plan*. A handful of these amino acids are very important to brain health, of which the three better known ones are:

Acetylcholine — transportation system, primary carrier of memory.

Serotonin and Norepinephrine — a lack of which affect mood, causing negative thoughts and depression.

Neurotransmitter shortages that cause depression and other mood disorders can often be reversed or improved by supplementing the concentrated nutrients:

Phosphatidyl Choline

Phosphatidyl Serine

Acetyl L-Carnitine

Healthy neurotransmitters are dependent upon a good diet. Many need nutrients such as amino acids, vitamins and minerals for their manufacture. The nutrients above help to restore neurotransmitter functions.

Minor strokes in the brain (multi-infarct dementia)

These can also be treated by nutritional therapy, herbal and natural medicines, food supplements and exercises to increase blood flow to the brain, including breathing exercises that alleviate stress. Many conditions can be improved and even sometimes altered by nutritional means. Often, all that is needed is the will, co-operation and support of an Integrated Health System, whereby allopathic medicine and a full range of complementary therapies, including homeopathic medicine, work together to provide the finest possible treatment in both residential and nursing homes. This health system would extend to include carers looking after people who wish to stay in their own home.

Stress

The adrenal glands produce the hormones adrenalin and cortisol, which stimulate the 'fight or flight' response when we are confronted with a stressful situation. Excessive stress increases the production of cortisol, and excess cortisol accelerates ageing of the brain. Continuous, long-term stress can lead to atrophy of the hippocampus (Patrick Holford, *The Alzheimer's Prevention Plan*, 152). Here are some specific ways in which cortisol can contribute to and worsen the symptoms of Alzheimer's and dementia:

1. Cortisol interferes with the brain's supply of glucose, thereby depriving the brain of fuel. This makes new memories hard to lay down and existing memories hard to retrieve.

2. Cortisol interferes with the brain's neurotransmitters that carry your thoughts.

3. Cortisol causes an excessive influx of calcium into brain cells, and over a long period of time creates free-radical molecules, which cause brain cells to dysfunction and eventually die. Billions of neurons die and millions more are badly damaged.

The solution is to avoid too much stress in your life.

Stress is a fact of life, and a small amount is actually good; it can motivate us to action, give us the impetus to make necessary changes in our lives and move forward in a creative way. However, too much stress leads to rapid ageing and will eventually lead to degenerative diseases, including those of the brain that become irreversible. Reducing stress improves circulation by lowering blood pressure. It is not the actual stresses in life that present the problem; they are not the cause. The cause can be an inability to adapt to a stressful situation, for example, in a stressful situation two people will react differently.

Continuous stress can also create certain nutritional deficiencies. Below are the symptoms of some possible deficiencies:

Vitamin B12 — may result in many symptoms, including psychotic behaviour, indifference, irritability, exhaustion and lack of energy.

Vitamin B1 — may result in the inability to learn anything new. There can also be symptoms of anxiety, obsessive thinking, confusion and memory loss.

Folic acid — may show symptoms of senility or dementia.

Zinc — it is estimated that fifty per cent of the population are zinc deficient. Zinc deficiency allows the body to absorb the aluminium contained in so many of today's products: from cooking pans, foil and drinking water, to aspirin, antacids and baking powder. Aluminium has been found through numerous studies to be linked to Alzheimer's disease.

Circulation

Impaired circulation affects the body and also the mind. Decreased blood flow brings about a slow degeneration of the brain as neurons gradually die. We now know that what is good for the heart is good for the head, and that maintaining good circulation is vital for the health of the brain. Neurons killed by the over-production of cortisol and other negative factors will impede blood flow to the brain's healthy neurons, thereby increasing memory loss and producing concentration problems. See page 37 for a simple exercise that will improve circulation.

Conditions which mimic Alzheimer's and dementia

There are other substances, diseases and conditions that can attack the immune system and cause symptoms which mimic those of Alzheimer's and dementia, such as confusion, memory loss and disorientation:

Chemicals and pesticides

Chemotherapy

Radiation of all kinds

Candida albicans

Excess exposure to certain chemicals, pesticides and radiation place a strain over time on the effectiveness of the immune system.

Candida albicans is a yeast-like fungus that is naturally present in a healthy gut, and normally presents no problem and will do no harm. Overgrowth of candida albicans, however, affects the central nervous system and can mimic dementia in its symptoms: depression, lethargy, irritability, memory loss and an inability to concentrate.

In her book, *God Helps Those That Help Themselves*, Hanna Kroegar cites a study carried out in the USA in a mental institution where, out of 169 adults studied, 163 had candida albicans overgrowth. Hanna's cure for the condition of overgrowth is simple:

Take acidophilus and/or bifidis supplements (powder
form) before each meal (obtainable from BioCare.
See *References and resources*).

Use garlic daily (raw or capsule).

Take a vitamin A supplement for two weeks.

In addition, boost the immune system (see page 36),
avoid all yeast products, reduce alcohol intake and
avoid brewers yeast, raw mushrooms, chocolate and
sweets.

7. A nutritional approach — healthy body, healthy brain

I would like to present a proactive approach that, at the very least, offers everyone who wants to take steps to prevent Alzheimer's or dementia the opportunity to do so. There are also suggestions that will help to alleviate these conditions if they have already developed.

Like all illnesses, as already mentioned, prevention is better than cure. The following list of preventative measures is not exhaustive. I have already mentioned the importance of creating a positive attitude, however, there are a few basic and important guidelines:

1. Diet — as I have already explained in detail, diet and nutrition are essential for maintaining a healthy body and a healthy brain. This chapter contains practical advice on how to improve diet and nutrition in older people.

2. Water — drink sufficient water in order to avoid dehydration and constipation.

3. Exercise — walking, cycling, gardening, dancing, yoga and pilates — all these activities improve circulation to both the body and the brain, as well as increasing oxygen and lowering stress levels, which in turn give a sense of well-being.

4. Singing and making music — these are fun and joyful activities that will enhance breathing and consequently oxygen levels within the body and also improve memory: a good way to enhance social life!

Supplementation

What then can we do to reverse deficiencies, build a healthy immune system and protect against further damage? We can make sure that we are receiving adequate nutrition in our diet and start with a good supplementation programme, using only supplements produced from ethical companies (see *References and resources* for some of these companies) who source organic and the best quality products possible. A reliable company will have credentials showing a long-term, recognized research programme, a willingness to share the fruits of that research, a good labelling system and a nutritionist who understands the health supplements on offer. Such companies will have stood the test of time.

A word of caution before embarking upon any supplementation programme: consult your GP and nutritionist. This is especially important if taking medication.

Suggested supplements

Vitamin A — a powerful antioxidant that protects the membrane of brain cells, which are easily damaged by free radicals. It also helps the circulatory system.

B vitamins — these are the most important for the brain.

B12 — necessary for the nervous system and for effective brain function. Vegans and vegetarians need to ensure they are getting an adequate supply in order to avoid pernicious anaemia.

B6 — converts stored blood sugar into glucose, the brain's only fuel. Helps to protect blood vessels and therefore provides protection from heart attacks. Helps to improve memory and boosts the immune system. Reduces levels of homocysteine (a type of amino acid).

B1 (thiamine) — a powerful antioxidant that works with B6 and vitamin E to destroy radicals, and as the brain's fuel converts glucose into energy

Folic acid — relieves depression and enhances circulation in the brain; therefore especially valuable in vascular dementia. Psychiatric symptoms appear much higher in elderly people who have low folic acid levels. In one study, low folic acid levels increased the likelihood of dementia by 300%. Folic acid also breaks down homocysteine.

B3 (niacin) — helps to manufacture neurotransmitters. Converts carbohydrates to glucose and lowers cholesterol. Also has a calming effect.

B5 (pantothenic acid) — vital to the synthesis of the brain's primary memory neurotransmitter, acetycholine.

Vitamin C — the most powerful antioxidant in existence and especially important for synergizing the antioxidant potential of other nutrients. One of the finest nutrients for longevity. Also protects against cardiovascular disease by improving arterial function. Another benefit is reduction of cholesterol. Vitamin C as an antioxidant works effectively with the antioxidant Co-enzyme Q10.

Vitamin D — necessary for the absorption of calcium and assimilating vitamin A. Natural food sources are fish oils, nettles and sunshine.

Vitamin E — protects neurons from damage by free radicals and even has the ability to restore damaged neurotransmitter-receptor sites on neurons. It is not only able to prevent deterioration of the brain but can also help to reverse the condition. When taken with selenium, can improve mood and cognitive function. It is also an antioxidant that can decrease cholesterol by over forty per cent. Like vitamin C, vitamin E decreases the risk of heart attack and stroke.

Selenium — helps remove heavy metals such as mercury from the body.

In recent years, some researchers have found that people with the highest levels of vitamin C, beta-carotene and vitamin E in their blood score best in memory tests. Such research indicates that antioxidants improve circulation and reduce the risk of the brain becoming inflamed and damaged, in the same way that antioxidants help reduce the risk of heart disease. We can see from this that cardiovascular disease is deeply connected to problems associated with diseases of the brain and memory loss.

This naturally leads us to the kitchen ... In order to consume sufficient nutrients, avoid excess dietary fats and stay healthy, it is recommended that we eat:

Essential fatty acids (EFAs) (See chapter four of Holford's *Optimum Nutrition for the Mind* for suggested reading and details on this subject.)

Foods low in saturated fats

Linolenic acid (omega-6) and alpha linolenic acid
(omega-3) — found in oily fish such as mackerel and
sardines, algae and linseed for vegans and vegetarians

Complex, wholegrain carbohydrates

Good quality protein

Fruit and vegetables (should form two thirds of our diet)

Eat wholegrains that have not had the bran and endosperm
or germ removed. In their natural balanced state, wholegrains
are a rich source of fibre, vitamins and minerals, antioxidants
and phytonutrients. Along with plentiful fresh fruit and
vegetables, they help build a healthy immune system, can
reduce blood pressure and may lower the risk of heart disease
— healthy heart, healthy brain! Whole fibre-rich grains present
a natural way to obtain bran in the diet that will help prevent
constipation. Wholegrains include corn, millet, oats, rice, rye
and wheat used in our daily bread and cereals. It is better to
use organically grown grains to avoid chemical sprays and
pesticides used in other agricultural practices. There are many
general well-attested health benefits and interesting books
written on the subject (see *References and resources*).

Giving several small nutrient-rich meals through the day
can rectify the problem of poor assimilation of nutrients.

Key nutrients that are found in vegetables, such as
vitamins and minerals, can be given daily in soups and tasty
vegetable drinks using a stock base such as Vecon.

Live, probiotic goat, sheep or cow's yoghurt provides
acidophilus daily, which helps with the absorption of
nutrients and digestion.

Drinks using slippery elm, or slippery elm and mallow,
with a small spoon of honey, can soothe the digestive tract.
All these measures will improve assimilation.

Boosting the immune system

To strengthen and boost the immune system, the following are all helpful:

Quaw Bark — taken in tincture form, it regenerates cells and improves production of red corpuscles.

Zinc — 10 mg a day (see page 28)

Herbs — a herbal combination of white pine bark, mugwort, myrrh, chamomile, catnip and mullein, marjoram tea, twice daily

Chaparral

Capsicum

Goldenseal

Echinacea

Pineapple

Papaya

Excellent herbal preparations can be obtained from the herbalist Jill Davies, Herbs Hands Healing (see *References and resources*).

Supplementation is best and likely to be more effective when carried out by a qualified nutritionist who understands the nutritional needs of older people. As a general guideline, the elderly better assimilate liquid tinctures and supplements in powder form. Reputable suppliers, some of which are listed at the back of the book, offer a free advisory service.

8. Brain gym exercises

Exercises that increase blood flow to the brain also improve cognitive function and stimulate the endocrine (hormone) system, which supplies the blood with substances that influence the activity of cells. The pineal gland produces calming melatonin and therefore, amongst other benefits, lowers stress levels.

In each of the following exercises, sit comfortably, with your spine straight and your arms relaxed and by your sides. Breathe in as you raise your arms, and out when you lower them.

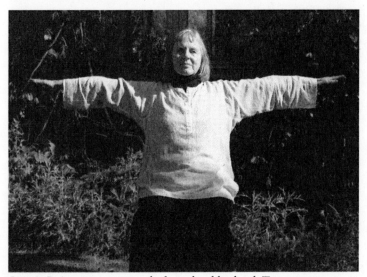

Step 1. Raise arms, outstretched, to shoulder level. Tense your arms and hands.

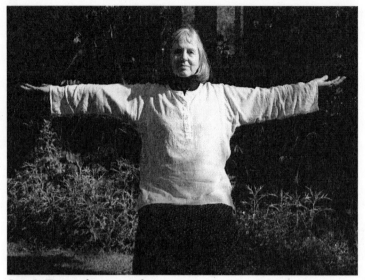

Step 2. Turn palms upward.

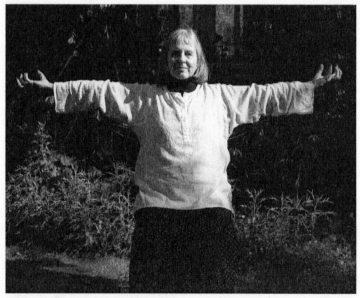

Step 3. Still tensed, form claw action with fingers.

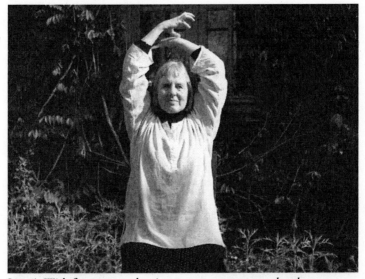

Step 4. With fingers tensed, raise your arms over your head.

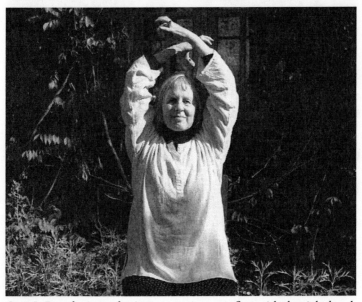

Step 5. Breathe in, and raise your arms; cross first with the right hand in front of the left; lower arms to shoulder level, breathing out; then repeat, crossing this time with the left hand forward. Continue the rhythm for as long as is comfortable — one to three minutes.

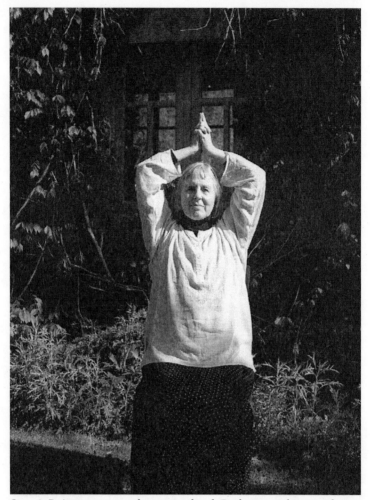

Step 6. Raise your arms above your head. Push your palms together.
Breathe normally, and hold for as long as is comfortable.

Now relax, and breathe deeply for a few minutes.

9. The art of converting a Zimmer frame into a hockey stick

For an elderly person suffering from Alzheimer's or dementia, the ideal way to spend the final years of life would be in their own home surrounded by loved ones and all that is familiar. This ideal state would depend upon a responsive 'care package' which offered professional help when needed in one's own home. In reality, this ideal situation is not possible for many families and they look for a residential care home where they can trust the manager and staff to look after their loved one as they would be looked after at home. From the many interviews and research programmes conducted, it is apparent that all is not well in the private sector. Residential homes are increasingly driven by profit, or put under pressure through too little government help, resources and consequent staff shortages. This can lead to low morale and little motivation to care beyond everyday personal needs. Too little emphasis and time is given to mobility, or to the necessary social and spiritual needs of the residents.

A familiar comment, often voiced by residents who find they are sitting for hour after hour, is, 'The trouble here is there is nothing to do; everything is done for you.' The future prospect of endless hours, days, months and often years stretching long and empty before them, without any seeming purpose, is daunting and can lead to depression, causing both mental and physical deterioration. Why should people make the effort to get out of bed and walk if there is no purpose or meaning to the day? As one resident woefully told me, 'I'm no use to man nor beast!'

For people no longer in their own homes, where there would have been plenty to occupy and interest them, addressing this commonly experienced problem requires creative and imaginative thinking. For people with Alzheimer's or dementia it forms a major role in enabling the brain to form new pathways and to compensate for what has been lost.

Recent research has discovered that the brain is sufficiently flexible to enable it to grow new dendrites (the branched projections of a neuron) that make it possible to regenerate connections in the brain for as long as we live. It is vital, therefore, that activities which stimulate the brain are undertaken in the early stages of Alzheimer's and dementia, since these forge new memories. On the other hand, inactivity and a sedentary lifestyle impede the laying-down of new memories.

As previously stated, dementia affects each individual in a different way. However, most would benefit from carrying out simple activities with their hands, such as folding paper napkins ready for the next meal, sorting laundry into socks, shirts, dresses etc. For those more able residents there are many more creative jobs to do around any home: arranging flowers into vases and containers; painting colours and shapes with large paintbrushes on to A3 sheets of paper and displaying the results of their efforts. Having a large basket of various musical instruments that residents can pick up and shake or tap as music is played can help to maintain physical co-ordination and awaken interest. Singing encourages deep breathing and is a joyful activity.

In place of negative thinking, which allows no real life or improvement for a person with dementia, we must focus on the capacity of the brain to form new pathways. All is not lost when brain cells deteriorate and die. But to form new pathways requires the will and resources of all those who care for older members of our society — to stimulate those in their care and enable them to achieve the best quality of life possible.

The people who now need our help come from an age when most would have started work from the age of thirteen or fourteen and worked until the age of sixty or sixty-five, some even older. In their earlier working lives, they would have worked long hours: at least a five-to-six day, forty-five hour week, with only one or occasionally two weeks holiday a year. With few modern-day conveniences, such as washing machines and vacuum cleaners, work around the house would have been physically harder and taken much longer.

Having thus spent so much of their working lives, to now find themselves cast out on a lonely and uncharted ocean with nothing to do — even worse, an ocean of people whom they have never met or chosen as companions — the experience is an anathema to many residents in homes. The situation must be daunting, and it is easy to become rudderless with no means of navigation other than reliance on the intelligence and empathy of care staff. So we can understand how important it is that close relatives and friends of the vulnerable loved one ensure that the residential home provides daily activities and facilitates effective social interaction.

Sudden enforced inactivity, after the initial pleasure in having everything done for them as if they're on holiday staying in a hotel, soon results in physical and mental deterioration. For people with Alzheimer's and dementia, who are already confused and distressed, this can result in increased stress levels, which further affect their behaviour. Keeping busy with activities, entertainment, and the comfort of having something to do, can help to ameliorate subsequent behavioural problems.

We recently heard a programme on the radio about Doritt Hoflight who is ninety-six years old. Having spent a lifetime as a researcher at Harvard Computers in the USA, Doritt is still working. She has an office at Yale, where she is working on research and producing the 'Bright Star Register.' She said with a laugh, 'I'm so busy, I don't have time to die!'

Nearer to home, we have learnt of a man who lives in Dorset, who was 104 years old in 2007. Remarkably, this man's career as a professional gardener has spanned ninety-three years. Mr Webber was forced to retire in 2006 because of painful arthritis in his knees, however, up until that time he worked most days of the week as a jobbing gardener and cared for six gardens around the village where he lived. Since retirement Mr Webber can only manage his own half-acre plot where he lives with his daughter. He reads, mostly without spectacles, but needs them for driving, and last I heard, his driving licence was valid until 2008!

A lady living nearby in East Devon is 101 years old, and persists in taking her daughter for punishing walks along the sea front. She started learning to play the guitar at the age of ninety, and still plays with nimble fingers.

These are just a few of the many true stories of remarkable people with very positive attitudes and the will to 'live' rather than to simply 'exist.'

10. A new life in a residential home — Shangri-la or Custer's Last Stand?

In this section, I discuss how we can change the experience of entering a residential home from 'Abandon hope, all ye who enter here!' to 'Welcome to your third age: new friends, new beginnings!'

Some people suffering from Alzheimer's or dementia have families who are able to offer care, either by adapting their own homes or by helping those who would prefer to continue living in their own home. In ideal circumstances, we remain surrounded by family and friends. The question is: how are those of us who don't have this level of family or friendly support going to live a fulfilled life and remain positive if we are unable to cope with day-to-day living? If we have to move into a nursing or residential home, how can we retain a positive and purposeful attitude, to avoid becoming depressed and institutionalized?

Before discussing the beneficial experiences of moving into a residential home, we will look at some feelings that are common to many people when they face the reality of moving home. Problems that arise after entering a residential home do not necessarily manifest straight away. There can be a gradual dawning of the situation in which the new resident finds himself or herself, which can produce symptoms of shock. This is especially prevalent with people suffering from Alzheimer's and dementia, whose likely emotions are:

Grief and loss — loss of home, family, friends, pets.

Frustration — doors locked; no longer able to go out without asking permission, or able to leave the building at all when in an EMI home.

Fear — no familiar faces; unable to find the toilet or familiar belongings.

Confusion — where am I? Why am I here? I want to go home. Where is my husband/wife/mother/ children?

Anxiety — incontinence and being toiletted, often by many different care staff; ladies toiletted by male carers can be a daily source of stress and embarrassment.

Depression — the realisation that no Prince or Princess Charming is going to rescue you, take you home or even out, without bringing you back again; the knowledge that your long past has gone, leaving an empty space each day with nothing to fill the gap.

Hopelessness — no freedom; no purpose

Even with people around that have knowledge and understanding of the condition, the mental pain of losing one's faculties has to be experienced to know what it is like. With dementia, as the condition develops, a person can feel distressed and ashamed because of perceived stigma; they can grow silent and depressed, caught in the fear of their condition and an empty future ahead. Who will listen? Who can understand? A common everyday expression, often uttered by sufferers at times of incredulity, is, 'I was speechless.' The experience of Alzheimer's and dementia frequently renders a person 'speechless' and for reasons other than the death of brain cells! I have often experienced the following reactions:

Speechless with fear

Speechless in the face of hopelessness

Speechless at the reactions of those around them

Speechless with anger

Sometimes this condition alternates with angry verbal outbursts, and even violence, until the time comes when the person speaks no more. Sadly, this is all too common.

Clearly there are people who enter residential homes to whom the above does not apply. With each person, it is a question of degree. However, many carers, relatives and friends will have experienced, as I have, one or more of the above emotions, and seen them work a devastating effect upon their loved one. The situation can be distressing and difficult to resolve. Anti-depressant drugs are not the answer; at best, they only offer temporary relief. Homeopathic remedies and herbal medicines can be effective, and along with good, ongoing management by well-trained and understanding staff, are now recognized as a much more safe, effective and creative approach.

We will now look at the above situations to see if there is a way of easing the pain and isolation experienced when moving into residential care.

Imagine what it would be like to leave the home you have lived in, often for many years, never to return again. Consider the emotions of grief and loss. No more will you do ordinary, everyday things: dust the mantle-shelf or put the cat out, make a cup of tea, telephone a friend, or wander into the garden and pluck a flower for the vase. The ordinary and simple everyday actions of life are gone. How would you feel? Worse, you are in a strange, hotel-like place, and you are told that this is now your home. Perhaps you do vaguely remember that this is not the place familiar to you as home. In that case, why do smiling faces reassure you that it *is* now your home and that you have already been told about this new 'home,' when you have no memory of ever being told? You are confused, yet the people seem friendly and nice. But where are the family, the cat or dog and the children? Panic and fear set in.

Such a reaction is quite common for people with Alzheimer's or dementia on first entering a residential or nursing home. To help a person who is fearful and confused needs one-to-one mentoring for as long as necessary to help them acclimatize to their surroundings. This would include making friends with compatible residents: discussing mutual memories of school, home, films and playing and singing music of their time; discussing likes and dislikes and playing simple games together. Hopelessness can only exist if there is no hope. A well-trained, understanding and skilled carer can show that this new phase of life can be interesting, if different. So much depends on the level of commitment and interaction of the carer, the other residents, and frequent visits and outings (if appropriate) by family and friends.

This level of care is seldom possible given the present-day funding and staffing levels in most homes, as it is incompatible with the drive for profit. Residents have to pay a heavy price to ensure one-to-one quality care. In a world where most assessments are made on cost-effectiveness, clearly a home that provided twenty-four-hour help of the highest quality would need extra resources and funding.

For care staff endeavouring to provide good and dignified care, remembering one of these two mnemonics — GET and SET — will greatly help. They stand for:

Glasses, Ears, Teeth
Spectacles, Ears, Teeth

These are terribly important to human dignity, orientation, communication, digestion, physical, mental and emotional health and well-being. So often in care homes, people are without their glasses, hearing aids or false teeth. This means they are unable to read or see other people clearly, hear when they are spoken to, or digest their food properly, which leads to health problems, loss of weight and constipation.

There are many reasons why spectacles, hearing aids and false teeth go missing, and each care home will have its own story to tell of weird and wonderful hiding places where GET have been discovered. However, if all care staff are trained to understand the prime importance of these aids to people in their care, they will ensure that each resident always has these personal items on them and check at regular intervals during the day. For those of us who have no need of false teeth, spectacles or a hearing aid, it requires imagination to understand how it must be for people dependent upon these aids.

To be unable to hear isolates us from the rest of the community because we can't understand or communicate. To be unable to see is a frightening situation, especially when voices and people are unfamiliar and surroundings are strange. And to be without teeth robs a person of their dignity, apart from being unable to masticate and therefore to digest food, which leads to a subsequent deterioration of health. All three of these situations can lead to depression that in turn will increase mental, physical and emotional deterioration. In any care home it cannot be beyond human ingenuity to devise a system whereby regular checks are made throughout the day to ensure that all residents are using their aids.

Nursing Homes .

A word on nursing care: my mother, Ruby, reached a stage in her condition after nine years of residential care when she needed nursing and was moved to a nursing home. She receives excellent round-the-clock care. However, nursing staff in nursing homes, as in hospitals, are not trained in the care of patients with Alzheimer's or dementia. I have already had the comment addressed to me that my mother would not know whether or not she was in bed or sitting out in her chair! It is an assumption that we cannot possibly know for certain. I will give an example. In my mother's previous residential EMI home, my husband Glyn and I used to take another resident with advanced dementia on outings with my mother. This lady for many years had only spoken incoherent sentences, to put it kindly, and we used to enter her world of 'gobbledegook' and try to make sense of it! However, one day at a local mill where we had gone for tea, we were standing on a small wooden bridge looking at the mill wheel and race, when this lady turned to us and said slowly, in perfect Queen's English, 'Do you know, I never thought that I would ever see this again.' There are many other experiences that echo this one, and demonstrate that as family, friends and carers, we should keep an open mind about what people with dementia do or do not understand.

Just as a baby or very young child cannot communicate preferences or needs through the medium of speech, neither can elderly EMI patients in the latter stages of their illnesses. Being able to anticipate and understand their unspoken needs is vital. Sitting in a comfortable chair is preferable to lying in bed, where deterioration can be rapid!

Feeding, too, can present problems, and all care staff attending to these duties should be trained in how to communicate effectively and offer meals in a slow, attentive and unhurried manner. My mother no longer speaks, yet I sometimes glean understanding in her eyes. I do, therefore, speak to her about everyday events and past shared experiences, including humorous exploits! Expressions, movement, gestures and even mood can convey thoughts and feelings. Most of us express the emotions of irritation, impatience, stress and anger (to name but a few) throughout our lives, as well as joy and happiness, without necessarily uttering a word. It takes skill to read this silent language. When helping a vulnerable person without recourse to speech, we can have an effect for good or ill.

11. Residential care — new homes, new thinking

The above paints a somewhat bleak picture for both prospective relatives and people who may one day find it necessary to enter a residential home. Yet we can make a difference in most areas that need change.

Funding — put pressure on the government through local MPs and support bodies such as The Alzheimer's Society and Help the Aged, who are also trying to bring about a change in policy.

Activities — become involved with a local residential or nursing home, either as a visitor or friend and engage residents in conversation.

Ideally a residential home should be homely. That means small enough to feel like home and not a hotel, with plenty of room to move about, but not too spacious. The best design could be an open-plan layout, preferably on one level, with plenty of inglenooks and a couple of lounges in which people with different needs can relax. Small really is beautiful, especially when one is old and vulnerable.

The first priority for any residential or nursing home is *training*. Staff who have not been specifically trained to care for the elderly and mentally infirm are in danger of responding in a damaging and inappropriate way to an already very vulnerable resident. Professional training in Alzheimer's and dementia care should be carried out by specialists in psychiatry, with practical hands-on experience of working with Alzheimer's and dementia. During training, each new carer should be supervised in the residential or nursing home until confident and competent in their work. A carer's work should be valued, seen as a vocation, command respect and a good salary. Building trust between management, carer and resident cannot be overemphasized. When trust is established and maintained as a way of life, then everyone blossoms and feels secure.

Further basic requirements for any residential or nursing home should be: a full-time physiotherapist or music and movement therapist to keep residents mobile; an occupational therapist, and a full-time activities organizer. At present, the provision of such care is optional and therefore at the mercy of the manager and owner of the home. They decide whether or not they wish to employ these types of care staff based on their budget and projected profit. It is scandalous that our National Health Service only funds basic care, and ignores the mental and emotional needs of older, vulnerable members of our society.

Anthroposophical medicine

No work on health would be complete without mentioning the immense service that anthroposophical (*anthropos* — man, and *sophia* — wisdom) medicine offers to those seeking an holistic and integrated approach to health and healing. This approach could help in understanding the conditions of Alzheimers' and dementia as well as in leading to their prevention. This integrated approach uses homeopathic, plant-based medicines as well as rhythmical massage and a range of artistic therapies, which take each individual need into account. It sees nutrition as part of the healing process. Dr Rudolf Steiner (1861–1925) developed this integrative approach to medicine along with Dr Ita Wegman, who opened clinics in Switzerland and Germany as early as 1921.

In an article in *New View* magazine, Summer 2007, Branc Zilavec drew attention to Steiner's lecture on Nutrition in Health and Illness, in which he referred to early Arabian physicians who believed every digestion was regarded as a partial illness. As a result, one eats oneself ill and digests oneself well again, thus healing takes place. Dr Steiner said:

> This view, which was in fact held for some time … is altogether something quite sound, because there exists no real borderline between what today is called 'eating oneself well' and 'eating oneself ill.' Just think how easily things can be disrupted by eating. Something that normally can be overcome quickly passes over into something that can no longer be overcome. Then one becomes ill. But the borderline between these two states really cannot be drawn at all.

Branc Zilavec goes on to say:

> If a person is constantly repeating a pattern of too much wrong choice, of bad quality foods day after day, then he or she will sooner or later — depending on an individual's constitutional strength — develop an illness …

As I've mentioned before, dementia means we lose the ability to direct the will 'to do' anything in the same way any more. A good analogy would be to a captain on a ship who has lost the rudder. There is a loss of self-awareness and functioning of normal mental and critical faculties. Nutrition plays a crucial role in ensuring that the physical body offers the mind the best blood supply possible to enable it to function at optimum levels.

In 2007 Radio 4's *The Food Programme* featured Dr Walter Yellowlees talking about the importance of good wholefood nutrition, and how we grow and resource our food. Dr Yellowlees, a retired GP now in his healthy nineties, was a breath of fresh air for common sense in a world where diets expounding this or that food, and claims and counterclaims urging us to eat this or not to eat that, abound. Dr Yellowlees has written a book of his experiences as a general practitioner in the Highlands of Scotland, called *Doctor in the Wilderness*. I can thoroughly recommend his book, in which he advocates sound nutrition using wholesome and unrefined foods in the prevention of disease. As he states:

> We know enough with our earthly senses to conclude that dietary faults are the main causes of the diseases mentioned in this book.

That thesis, I believe, is also true for diseases of the brain. Doctor Yellowlees reminded me of an old and very true saying: 'We are just as old as our arteries.'

So why bother about a very old person who is coming to the end of their life, and to all intents and purposes is at the best quietly incomprehensible, or at the worst bothersome or even aggressive? Apart from the obvious benefits to us of showing love and compassion, what if the life of that person is important for the whole of humankind? Dr Rudolf Steiner certainly believed that to be the case, as he stated during a conversation with a lady who was moved by pity for a very old and sick person who lay paralysed in bed. This lady said that it might be better if the sick woman was released. Dr Steiner answered very earnestly, 'No, every hour she lives on earth is important for the whole of mankind.' Furthermore, Steiner stated:

> And so when Kant had grown old and demented,
> he had grown glorious rather than demented for the
> world of the spirit.

I am not alone in my interpretation of Dr Steiner's comments: that the more we try to understand what people with senile dementia offer the rest of humanity, and show true compassion and love, the more we will understand what their mission and ours on earth may be. It can be stated more simply as creative development, through our search for meaning and understanding of the very essence of our being. Dr Pieper-van den Berg, MD, described the process as follows:

> We can divide the path from birth to death into four
> parts. The first twenty-one years are years of gathering
> physical energies, powers of soul, powers of mind and
> spirit. At twenty-one we are ready for the world and
> able to offer all these abilities, with the delicate turning
> point in the middle, between thirty and thirty-three
> years of age. The third stage of life brings questions
> and doubts. One feels the need to change everything,
> to be more free and independent. Anxieties, pride
> and too great an opinion of self have to be dealt with.
> After the age of fifty we can face the task of getting
> more independent in our habits, developing the art of

life, grow calmer and perhaps find a new relationship to religion. And finally, we need to become truly social, independent of physical infirmities, to feel love for other human beings, be mild in our judgements, for this alone will make communion possible in the world.

A new challenge

The courage to take new thinking and practices into the twenty-first century is a challenge to every residential home, and yet offers an opportunity to demonstrate that growing older, even if that means entering a home, can be a rewarding and healthy experience. Success or failure will depend upon a strong desire on the part of the owners, managers and staff to understand and accept the vital importance of both *food* and *activity* as healing therapies. Furthermore, that it is possible to maintain a healthy body and a healthy mind into advanced old age. The soup recipes included in the final section of this book are not only delicious and varied but have been chosen for their nutritional qualities, and provide the daily vitamins, minerals and fibre necessary for a healthy immune system and general good health.

Also important to health is a feeling of happiness and of belonging. This can be achieved in part by encouraging a daily safe and appropriate involvement in the running of the home and garden. Joy and fun are infectious: if staff are happy and fulfilled in their work, then this type of infection is one that the residents will gladly catch! To provide such a happy environment in which the resident feels truly 'at home,' secure, fulfilled and happy is a state, I suggest, that we would all like to attain, accepting off-days as a reality of life.

Remember that we may have to enter a home ourselves one day. We all wish to reach this special time of our lives in sound mind, but increasing evidence and present trends indicate that unless we take preventative measures, many of us will suffer serious mental decline — Alzheimer's disease or one of the many forms of dementia. For the majority of people who adopt a healthy lifestyle, *this need not happen.* And even those who will suffer from these conditions can, with the right help and positive attitudes, live and enjoy a good quality of life.

Until funding increases, one aim of this book is to offer practical and workable suggestions to nursing staff, and to all carers, that can be used at minimum cost in the home or in residential homes. I aim to propose a positive approach to ageing, which does not deny the ageing process but acknowledges that a good quality of life can be achieved and maintained. I also offer a challenge to residential and nursing homes to put these suggestions to the test. They can judge for themselves whether or not their implementation will bring about improved mental and physical health and well-being among their residents.

12. The cost of funding a new approach

We clearly need government support and a good financial structure in order to offer better health care, care at home and quality residential and nursing care. Excellent help and care packages exist for families and young children, those with special needs and for those on low incomes. Now we need the government to recognize the needs of a generation who contributed many years of labour to this country, many of whom survived a pre-war recession, a world war and its hardship, and who all deserve a high quality of care in their own hour of need.

In order to provide this quality of care, extra government funding is vital. But it also involves a cost that moves beyond monetary considerations: that of teaching present and future generations of young people that, if we simply do not care what happens to older people, we are fostering an attitude of disregard, disrespect and discrimination.

Along with increased funding there is a need for the government and all professionals involved to have the will to approach these potentially debilitating conditions with a positive and creative attitude. This means the will to carry out research that is open minded enough to look at every aspect of the condition and use treatments, therapies and activities that work to bring about an improvement. Unless we grasp the nettle now to bring about change, in this affluent and educated twenty-first century, then we are hardly more enlightened than our well-documented nineteenth-century ancestors, with their often inhumane attitudes and institutions!

There are enormous benefits to be gained for all involved by working together to seek ways to improve nutrition, therapies and activities, and hence improve the quality of life for people suffering from these conditions. For carers working with people with Alzheimer's and dementia to see an improvement, however small, in the well-being of people in their care, would immensely increase their job satisfaction.

Practical suggestions at minimal cost

I would now like to look at a few practical, yet simple, ways that can, with *minimal* cost, be introduced to implement nutritional and occupational change in care homes:

- Daily soups and juices to provide adequate and digestible vitamins and minerals; slippery elm and live yoghurt to aid assimilation.
- Plentiful filtered or mineral water for residents to drink to avoid dehydration.
- Liquid or powdered supplements, when appropriate and agreed with your GP.
- One-to-one conversations and activity within a small group.
- Physiotherapy; music and movement therapy; deep-breathing exercises.
- Daily occupational therapy in small groups.
- Games to improve dexterity, such as 'catch' with a soft ball.

'Past times' discussions, using artefacts appropriate
for the age group — ideally a room set aside for
memorabilia.

Supervised 'help' — household and gardening tasks,
with staff.

Weekly outings to places of interest, including tea out.

Musical entertainment and singing.

Hymn singing on Sundays to allow residents who
are no longer able to attend church to partake in a
spiritual activity.

Frequent GET (Glasses, hearing aid, false teeth) checks.

Visits from local schools to sing, dance, read poems or
plays and converse.

Family, friends and volunteer visits to sing, chat and
have fun.

True costs and benefits

In these days of measuring cost-effectiveness, a healthy and
happy old age will considerably reduce NHS bills and the
necessity for drugs, give managers and care staff a more
enjoyable and less stressful environment in which to work,
and effect positive interaction through the increased well-
being of their residents.

In the short term, these changes can immeasurably improve
quality of life, which is especially vital to the increasing
number of people who already suffer from Alzheimer's and
dementia, and to their families.

In the long term, and if implemented, the changes suggested
in this book could revolutionize the current attitudes and
practices sometimes used in the present management of

Alzheimer's and dementia, and make entering a residential or nursing home a happy event rather than one of dread.

Of political interest will be the savings on NHS bills, especially the huge amount of money spent on pharmaceutical drugs and hospitalization. Instead of the gloom and doom forecasts of how older people represent a terrible drain on national resources and constitute 'bed blocking,' people living motivated, healthier and more mobile lives will save millions of pounds spent now unnecessarily on drugs and hospitalization.

13. A final word

To the person with Alzheimer's or dementia, the present is all they have on which to hang their whole existence. The present encompasses the past — a vivid panorama of memories and longings of family, friends, pets, places visited, experiences — all jumbled into the *now* and all very real. Often the memory of past days is so 'present' and real that it causes distress: the person feels they have to 'fetch the children from school,' 'get Mother's dinner' or 'catch the bus,' and endless other concerns from the past. Of course, we, the carers, know that the 'children' are now in their fifties and sixties, Mother has long since passed away, and the needed bus is in another town and from another time.

However, the immediate situation has to be handled with care and sensitivity, the drama entered into and taken into another scene and ending. These are situations that people who care for someone with Alzheimer's or dementia have to deal with daily. What matters is that this very real, long-gone past is listened to, taken seriously as the situation arises, and then taken forward with assurance and reassurance that all will be well. To challenge and confront a person's present reality in the pursuit of objective truth causes untold stress, because 'fetching the children from school,' or whatever the crisis of the moment may be, *is* true for the person with Alzheimer's or dementia.

From my fifteen years of personal experience and observation, the secret is to enter in imagination into their 'real' world, listen to the story unfolding, even albeit in a garbled form, then reassure in a way appropriate for the individual. From there it is possible to move into something pleasant to do — perhaps making a cup of tea together. In that way, the future is brought into the present without fuss or stress.

For each individual entering this unknown and frightening world of confusion, loss of memory and intellect, with many faculties and physical bodily functions failing, there is no preparation. As with death, few of us ever consider the reality or possibility that one day we may suffer from the condition and make preparations. How can we?

In the future I hope we can extend our present knowledge and understanding, and work creatively with what we know, to prevent the conditions of Alzheimer's and dementia.

What then,
Shall we sit idly down and say,
'The night hath come; it is no longer day?'
Something remains for us to do or dare;
Even the oldest tree some fruit may bear;
For age is opportunity no less
Than youth itself, though in another dress,
And as the evening twilight fades away
The sky is filled with stars invisible by day.

Henry Wadsworth Longfellow

Recipes for super soups

The future belongs to those nations who are willing and capable to adopt the science of nutrition, and take full advantage of its teachings.

Dr G von Wendt (Sweden)

The following represent a small sample of nutritional soups that I have chosen to ensure that older people receive the vitamins and minerals necessary for good health and are able to digest and assimilate the nutrients.

The golden rule to aid health and digestion is to use very low heat when sautéing vegetables and to use olive oil or small amounts of stock in preference to any saturated fats. Having said that, the occasional use of butter for the benefit of enhanced taste with certain soups and dishes is preferable than using other saturated fats or oils.

At the end of each recipe you will find a short paragraph showing relative food values. This has been added to help you choose appropriate ingredients for a soup, for example when colds, coughs and influenza are around and it would be helpful to know which vegetables and herbs can aid the healing of these conditions. This can be particularly helpful in a residential home.

Quantities in each recipe are for six people — adjust according to number.

Onion, garlic and carrot soup

Ingredients

1½ pt (700 ml) rich stock or organic stock cube
4 medium onions
4 garlic cloves
1 lb (450 g) carrots
1 tsp turmeric
handful fresh parsley or 1 tsp dried

Method

• Dry roast the turmeric in a thick-based pan for one minute.
• Add a small amount of stock (1 in/2½ cm) and bring to the boil.
• Add onions and garlic; simmer for 1 minute.
• Add carrots; simmer for 20 minutes.
• Add herbs; simmer for a further 5 minutes.
• Liquidize.
• Garnish with fresh parsley.

Nutritional value

Onions contain vitamins A, B, C and E, calcium, iron, magnesium, potassium, bioflavanoids. An onion contains natural antiseptic oils similar to garlic, which are anti-microbial. Onions help reduce blood pressure, prevent blood clots from forming and lower blood sugar levels. Onions increase the flow of urine and aid digestion as well as acting as a decongestant if you are sufferings from a cold or blocked sinuses. Both arthritis and rheumatism are relieved because of reduced inflammation.

Garlic can help to reduce blood pressure and heart disease. Garlic is also good for colds, especially when combined with ginger, and helps clear bronchitis. Garlic contains a powerful antiseptic, and in the Middle Ages people wore cloves around their necks to protect them from the plague (see also recipe for *Onion winter warmer*).

Carrots are a powerful antioxidant and immensely rich in carotene (provitamin A), B3, C and E, folic acid, sodium, calcium, potassium, phosphorus and fibre. Carrots protect the lungs, liver and kidneys, and carotene is essential for healthy eyes. In clinics, raw carrot is widely used in the treatment of cancer, however, because of the heavy use of artificial fertilisers and pesticides, only use organic carrots.

Turmeric purifies the blood, strengthens digestion and improves liver function. It also kills harmful bacteria. Recent research shows that it has anti-tumour properties, and enhances memory.

Parsley is rich in vitamins and minerals, in particular A, B, C and E, iron, potassium, magnesium and copper. Parsley has many health properties that include helping to prevent anaemia, stimulating the appetite, alleviating constipation, dyspepsia and flatulence. It is best used raw as heating quickly destroys some of the effective properties.

Carrot, dill and coriander soup

Ingredients
2 pt (1 l) vegetable stock
1 large onion
2 garlic cloves
2 lb (900 g) carrots
1 tsp ground coriander
1 oz (30 g) fresh coriander
1 oz (30 g) fresh dill
yoghurt for garnish

Method

- Dry roast the coriander in heavy-based pan for 1 minute.
- Add 1 dessertspoon of olive oil; warm gently.
- Sauté the onions and crushed garlic.
- Add the carrots.
- Simmer for 25 minutes.
- Add the chopped coriander and dill in the last 5 minutes.
- Serve with yoghurt.

Nutritional value

Carrots are a powerful antioxidant and immensely rich in carotene (provitamin A), B3, C and E, folic acid, sodium, calcium, potassium, phosphorus and fibre. Carrots protect the lungs, liver and kidneys and carotene is essential for healthy eyes. In clinics, raw carrot is widely used in the treatment of cancer, however, because of the heavy use of artificial fertilizers and pesticides, only use organic carrots whenever using raw.

Dill contains vitamins A and C, calcium and potassium. Dill soothes upset stomachs, can stimulate a poor appetite, and helps in cases of flatulence.

Coriander contains vitamin B, folic acid and minerals, particularly potassium and calcium. Coriander helps relieve indigestion, especially abdominal pain, and constipation. Coriander has antibiotic properties too.

Courgette soup

Ingredients

2 tbsp olive oil
2 onions
4 cloves garlic
8 oz (225 g) courgettes

1 lb (450 g) tomatoes (fresh or tinned)
2 small potatoes
4 oz (100 g) fresh or frozen garden peas
2 pt (1 l) hot stock
6 leaves fresh basil
sea salt
freshly ground black pepper
1½ oz (40 g) curly pasta
optional: parmesan cheese

Method

- Warm the olive oil over a gentle heat and add the sliced onions and chopped garlic; cook until transparent.
- Add the sliced courgettes and cook for 10 minutes.
- Add the sliced (or tinned) tomatoes; cook until softened.
- Add the diced potatoes; simmer until nearly cooked.
- Add the peas, pasta and seasoning; simmer until cooked (about 10 minutes).
- Add the chopped basil and parmesan cheese (if included).
- Garnish with a few fresh basil leaves.

Nutritional value

Courgettes are high in vitamin C and also contain vitamins A and B, magnesium phosphorus, potassium and zinc. Courgettes can help bladder and kidney inflammation.

Fresh peas are extremely nourishing, being high in protein as well as carbohydrates and vitamins A, B and E. Peas also help anaemia and low blood pressure.

Tomatoes are a good source of vitamins A and C and are also high in fibre, potassium and folic acid. The acids (malic, citric and oxalic) activate silicon in the body that loosens stiff joints and therefore brings relief to chronic arthritis (rheumatoid) and rheumatism. (A note of caution: do not use green tomatoes or eat green parts of the plant as they contain poisonous alkaloids).

Basil is good for the digestion and is used to treat gastrointestinal problems.

Potatoes are a source of vitamin C (lost on storage) and potassium; the skins contain protein (see recipe for *Celery and potato soup*).

Beetroot and lemon soup

Ingredients

1 ½ pt (700 ml) stock
1 medium onion
2 cloves crushed garlic
4 medium beetroot
1 small red cabbage
1 medium parsnip
1 large carrot
1 stick celery
2 tomatoes or ½ small tin
1 dessert apple
1 dsp organic blackstrap molasses or molasses sugar
1 dsp lemon juice
a good handful chopped basil or 1 dsp dried basil

Method

- Gently sauté the chopped onion and crushed garlic until translucent.
- Add the thinly-sliced red cabbage and dessert apple, celery, molasses and lemon juice; cover with a lid.
- Cook for 5 minutes, shaking occasionally.
- Add the chopped carrot, parsnip and sliced beetroot.
- Add hot stock.

- Simmer for 30–40 minutes.
- Drizzle with yoghurt.

Nutritional value

Celery was once widely recommended for the treatment of rheumatism.

Beetroot is rich in potassium and fibre, and the leaves also contain vitamins A and C, iron, calcium, magnesium, potassium and other trace minerals, as well as bioflavonoids. Beetroot cleanses the liver, is excellent for the blood and circulation, and is used to treat anaemia. As well as being nutritious, it is easy to digest. Use both the leaves and root in soup.

Lemon is an important antioxidant, being rich in vitamin C and flavonoids, and will help fight infection and strengthen the immune system.

Parsnips are a good source of vitamins A and C, carbohydrate, potassium, calcium and fibre. They can help the digestion of people who are intolerant to milk, and in various types of digestive inflammation and irregularities.

Red cabbage is rich in vitamin C and contains many of the nutritional benefits of cabbage (see recipe for *Onion winter warmer*).

Organic, unsulphured blackstrap molasses contains some B vitamins and trace minerals that are beneficial to health and is rich in usable iron.

Celeriac and sweet potato soup

Ingredients
1 pt (500 ml) onion stock
1 medium celeriac
1 medium onion

1 clove garlic

2 sweet potatoes

2 medium potatoes

2 tsp turmeric

fresh or dried herbs and 6 sage leaves

Method

- Heat the turmeric in a dry, heavy-bottomed pan for 1 minute; shake.
- Add a small amount hot stock.
- Add the chopped onion; sauté until translucent.
- Add the sliced celeriac, sweet potatoes and potatoes.
- Simmer with the lid on for 1 minute.
- Add the rest of the stock; simmer for half an hour.
- Add the herbs in the last 5 minutes.
- Liquidize.
- Garnish with fresh parsley.

Nutritional value

Celeriac helps lower cholesterol and benefits the circulatory system. It contains vitamins A, B and C, potassium, magnesium and manganese.

Sweet potatoes contain considerable amounts of vitamin A, and also vitamins C and E and some protein. They are a richly antioxidant food that can help with conditions such as cancer. They are also rich in fibre.

Sage goes well with garlic. It has powerful antiseptic, expectorant and stimulant properties. Sage is also effective in clearing excess mucus from the lungs, and in a head cold. Sage is especially effective for sore throats. It also aids digestion.

Onion winter warmer

Ingredients
Small amount of stock
2 white and 2 large red onions
1 small head garlic (about 6–8 cloves)
2 leeks
3 carrots
4 large kale or dark cabbage leaves
1 bunch watercress
1 medium-sized apple
1 sprig rosemary
fresh marjoram or 1 tsp dried
fresh thyme or 1 tsp dried
fresh basil or 1 tsp dried
fresh mint or 1 tsp dried
walnut-sized piece of root ginger
1 tbsp organic blackstrap molasses
2 tsp arrowroot (or as packet instructions)

Method
- Heat a small amount of stock in a large saucepan.
- Add the onions, garlic and leeks and simmer for 5 minutes.
- Add the carrots and ginger and simmer 10 minutes.
- Add the cabbage leaves, watercress (saving sprigs for garnish), herbs, molasses and apple.
- Mix the arrowroot in cold water into a paste and stir it into the soup.
- Simmer for a further 20 minutes.
- Liquidize.
- Garnish with a few sprigs of watercress.

Nutritional value

This soup is excellent for relieving colds, coughs, influenza and bronchial conditions.

Onions contain vitamins B, C and E, carotene, calcium, iron, phosphorus, potassium, sodium, sulphur and traces of copper. Onions not only help colds and influenza, they are also antibiotic and anti-fungal, similar to garlic, which is antibiotic, anti-fungal and reduces cholesterol levels in the blood. Onions actively reduce blood pressure and blood sugar levels.

Garlic is excellent for cleansing the system of parasites; also for gastric conditions.

Leeks contain vitamins B and C, calcium, iron, magnesium, phosphorus, potassium, silica and sulphur. As with onions and garlic, leeks are excellent for the digestive tract, arthritis and for constipation, although not quite so active as both onions and garlic.

Kale or dark greens (that we all know from childhood from our parents urging us to eat up our greens) are, and have been recognized throughout history, as being extremely good for health. They are rich in vitamins A, B, C, K and E and in the minerals iron, potassium and calcium, and antioxidants.

Cabbage generally improves circulation by purifying the blood and the latest research shows that it can help prevent cancer. Other benefits are for asthmatic disorders, kidney and bladder problems and arthritis.

Watercress contains vitamins A, B, C, D and E, nicotinamide, and many trace minerals including manganese, iron, phosphorus, iodine, calcium, potassium, sodium and sulphur. Because of its many antibiotic properties it is a very useful preventative medicine, especially in congestive illnesses. Watercress is particularly effective for liver cleansing and helps arterial conditions, arthritis and rheumatism.

Organic, unsulphured blackstrap molasses contain some B vitamins and trace minerals that are beneficial to health and are rich in body-usable iron.

Apples contain many vitamins and minerals, sugars and enzymes that benefit the digestive system. Uncooked, they have an alkaline effect so are easily assimilated. They are, therefore, especially beneficial for older people. The malic and tartaric acid in apples aids digestion and supports liver function. Apples are excellent for numerous conditions including insomnia, catarrh, constipation, liver problems and worms. We can consider 'an apple a day' to truly prove an all-round health tonic!

Marjoram is helpful as an anti-spasmodic, expectorant and bactericide. It helps the healing process by increasing the number of white blood cells that fight infection. It is therefore especially effective for fighting colds, bronchitis and influenza. The digestive system is also stimulated by marjoram.

Thyme has antibacterial, anti-fungal, anti-spasmodic and expectorant properties, more powerful than those contained in marjoram. The above properties for marjoram apply, plus protection against intestinal, throat and bronchial infections.

Basil has anti-spasmodic and antiseptic properties and is used to ease stomach cramps, vomiting and constipation. It is also used to calm the nervous system and help with insomnia. Over the years it has commonly been used to treat whooping cough and head colds.

Spearmint is known to soothe and aid digestive problems including nausea, IBS (irritable bowel syndrome), indigestion and colitis. It is also useful in fighting colds, fevers and influenza.

Ginger is used to alleviate colds, influenza and stomach upsets because it induces sweating that cleanses the system.

Parsnip, leek and apple soup

Ingredients

1 large onion
2 leeks
3 medium-sized parsnips
1 large Bramley cooking apple
1 tbsp extra virgin, cold-pressed olive oil
1 pt (500 ml) stock
$\frac{1}{2}$ pt (250 ml) milk or soya milk
$\frac{1}{2}$ tsp powdered kelp
1 tsp mixed herbs
a good handful chopped parsley

Method

- Gently warm the oil in a large saucepan; sauté the vegetables and apple for 5 minutes, shaking frequently.
- Add the stock, kelp and herbs, retaining a little parsley for a garnish.
- Bring to boil and simmer for 30 minutes.
- Add the milk (or soya) then liquidize.
- Sprinkle with parsley and serve.

Nutritional value

Parsnips are a good source of vitamins A and C, carbohydrate, potassium, calcium and fibre. They can help the digestion of people who are intolerant to milk, and with various types of digestive inflammation and irregularities.

Leeks contain vitamins B and C, calcium, iron, magnesium, phosphorus, potassium, silica and sulphur. As with onions and garlic, leeks are excellent for the digestive tract, arthritis and for constipation, although they are not quite so active as both onions and garlic.

Parsley is rich in vitamins and minerals, in particular A, B, C and E, iron, potassium, magnesium and copper. Parsley has many health properties that include preventing anaemia, stimulating the appetite, alleviating constipation, dyspepsia and flatulence. It is best used raw as heating quickly destroys some of the effective properties.

Kelp, as with other seaweeds, is high in vitamins and minerals, especially iodine, and is a nourishing addition to soups. Kelp aids metabolism and nourishes the thyroid gland. It also helps ease catarrh, sore throats and coughs.

Pumpkin, spinach and sweet potato soup

Ingredients
1 medium onion
2 cloves garlic
1 lb (450 g) pumpkin
8 oz (225 g) spinach
2 sweet potatoes
3 tomatoes
1 tbsp extra virgin, cold-pressed olive oil
3 pt (1.5 l) vegetable stock
1 bay leaf
chives

Method
- Gently heat the oil in a large saucepan.
- Add the finely-chopped onion and sauté until transparent.
- Add the roughly-chopped pumpkin and sweet potatoes in bite-sized pieces.
- Add the chopped tomatoes.
- Bring slowly to the boil, and simmer on a low heat for 20 minutes until tender.

Add the finely-shredded spinach and simmer for 1 more minute.

Sprinkle over the chopped chives and season before serving.

Nutritional value .

Pumpkins contain antioxidant vitamins including folic acid. Pumpkins are low in calories and have a calming effect upon digestion. Pumpkins help relieve constipation, having a slightly laxative effect.

Spinach contains vitamins A, B, C and K, folic acid, and the minerals potassium, magnesium, iron, iodine and phosphorus. Popeye knew a thing or two — spinach is indeed good for you, especially if you are anaemic. This carotenoid contains lutein, which benefits the eyes. However, only allow spinach to cook for one minute as it yields up oxalic acid that binds the trace minerals, with the result that the high calcium and iron content cannot be properly utilized. The oxalic acid can be partially neutralized by adding yoghurt or milk. The most nutritious way to serve spinach is raw, so it's best chopped and added to the soup in the last minute of cooking time.

Bay leaves are good for the digestive system but also have anti-spasmodic and antiseptic properties.

Celery and potato soup

Ingredients

$1^{1}/_{2}$ pt (700 ml) stock
2 tsp turmeric
1 large onion
1 head celery
2 medium potatoes
1 oz (25 g) butter
2 fl oz (50 ml) milk

Method

- Shake the turmeric in a dry saucepan over a low heat for 1 minute, and continue shaking.
- Remove from the heat; add butter, the chopped vegetables, and gently sauté for 5 minutes, shaking frequently.
- Add the stock, cover and bring to the boil; simmer for 25 minutes.
- Add milk.
- When cool, blend in a liquidizer.
- Reheat slowly and season.

Nutritional value

Celery contains vitamins A, B and C, calcium, magnesium, manganese and potassium. Celery is easy to digest and helps in cases of poor digestion. Celery has an alkaline effect on the system, which benefits the skin. Celery is used in the treatment of both rheumatism and gout, but is also helpful for lowering high blood pressure, relieving catarrh and diarrhoea. Raw celery is good for a sore throat.

Potatoes contain vitamin C and potassium, although vitamin C levels will rapidly fall through long storage. The skin of the potato contains most of the nutrients: traces of carotene, vitamins B and C, and the minerals iron, phosphorus, calcium, potassium, sodium and sulphur.

Recent research has shown the effectiveness of turmeric for enhancing memory.

Vegetable broth

To be served as a mid-morning drink or as a 'cocktail' before lunch.

Ingredients

4 heads celery (keep heart for braising or salads)
3 medium onions
3 cloves garlic (crushed)
outer cabbage leaves (kale, spring greens, spinach etc.)
pea pods (if available)
3 leeks
3 raw carrots, grated
parsley (preferably fresh)
Yeastrel or Vecon

Method

• Wash all the vegetables, removing any damaged parts, and cut into small pieces without peeling.
• Place in a large saucepan, and just cover with cold water; put the lid on.
• Simmer for 45 minutes.
• Strain and add Yeastrel or Vecon.
• The strained vegetables can be liquidized and added to the soup.

Juiced vegetables and fruits provide a simple way to ensure older people are digesting the vital vitamins and minerals that their bodies need. Both professional and home juicers are available and are not costly.

There are many good recipe books that use both winter and summer vegetables and fruits. Herbal books also showing ways of using the many different herbs with health benefits (see recommendations in *References and resources*).

The above suggestions are by no means comprehensive or the last word on nutritious soups. To offer a more substantial soup, lentils, chickpeas, butter, kidney and haricot beans can all be added. Soak dried beans well and boil them vigorously for ten minutes before simmering to destroy an indigestible enzyme that is present, particularly in red beans. Pot or pearl barley is a good winter addition, and so are split peas.

References and resources

Alzheimer's Society (2003) *Great Minds Think Differently: New Frontiers in Alzheimer's Research*, Alzheimer's Society, London

Bennett, Peter (2002) *Writings on Nutrition and Behaviour*, The Restorative Health Company, Devon, www.rehealth.co.uk

Camps, Annegret; Hagenhoff, Brigitte & Van der Star, Ada (2008) *Anthroposophic Care for the Elderly*, Floris Books, Edinburgh

Cook, Wendy E. (2003) *Foodwise: Understanding What We Eat and How it Affects Us, the Story of Human Nutrition*, Clairview Books, East Sussex

Graimes, Nicola, *Vegetarian: The Greatest Ever Vegetarian Cookbook*, Hermes House, London

Hark, Lisa & Deen, Darwin (2006) *The Wholegrain Diet Miracle*, Dorling Kindersley, London

Holford, Patrick (2005) *The Alzheimer's Prevention Plan: 10 Proven Ways to Stop Memory Decline and Reduce the Risk of Alzheimer's*, Piatkus Books, London

—, (2003) *Optimum Nutrition for the Mind*, Piatkus Books, London

Khalsa, Dharma Singh & Stuath, Cameron (1999) *Brain Longevity: The Breakthrough Medical Program that Improves Your Mind and Memory*, Warner Books, New York

Koenig-Coste, Joanne (2003) *Learning to Speak Alzheimer's: The New Approach to Living Positively with Alzheimer's Disease*, Vermilion, London

Kroegar, Hanna (1984) *God Helps Those Who Help Themselves*, Hanna Kroeger Publications, Colorado

McVicar, Jekka (2004) *New Book of Herbs*, Dorling Kindersley, London

Steiner, Rudolf (1991) *Nutrition and Stimulants: Lectures and Extracts*, Biodynamic Farming and Gardening Association, Kimberton, USA

Van Bentheim, Tineke (2006) *Home Nursing for Carers*, Floris Books, Edinburgh

Van Straten, Michael (1999) *Superjuice: Juicing for Health and Healing*, Mitchell Beazley, London

Wolff, Dr Otto (1988) *Anthroposophical Medicine and its Remedies*, Tobias Therapeutic Publishing, South Africa

Yellowlees, Walter (2001) *A Doctor in the Wilderness*, Dr W. Yellowlees, Perthshire

Yutang, Lin (1998) *The Importance of Living*, HarperCollins Publishers, London

Waldemar, Gunhild & Burns, Alistair (2009) *Alzheimer's Disease (Oxford Neurology Library)*, Oxford University Press, Oxford

Alzheimer's Society

Devon House, 58 St Katharine's Way, London E1W 1JX, UK
Helpline: 0845 300 0336
Tel: +44 (0) 20 7423 3500
Fax: +44 (0) 20 7423 3501
Email: enquiries@alzheimers.org.uk
Website: www.alzheimers.org.uk
Living with Dementia, the Alzheimer's Society magazine

Laboratory intolerance and allergy testing

YorkTest Laboratories Ltd.
York Science Park, York YO10 5DQ, UK
Tel: 0800 074 6185 (UK only) or +44 (0) 1904 410410
Email: customercare@yorktest.com
Website: www.yorktest.com

Good-quality supplements

Higher Nature Ltd.
Burwash Common, East Sussex TN19 7LX, UK
Tel: 0800 458 4747
Email: info@higher-nature.co.uk
Website: www.highernature.co.uk

BioCare Ltd.
Lakeside, 180 Lifford Lane, Kings Norton, Birmingham,
West Midlands B30 3NU, UK
Tel: +44 (0) 121 433 3727
Email: biocare@biocare.co.uk
Website: www.biocare.co.uk

Weleda (UK) Ltd.
Heanor Road, Ilkeston, Derbyshire DE7 8DR, UK
Tel: +44 (0) 115 9448222
Email: sales@weleda.co.uk
Website: www.weleda.co.uk

Herbs, Hands, Healing Ltd.
Station Road, Pulham Market, Norfolk IP21 4XF, UK
Telephone 0845 345 3727
Email: info@herbshandshealing.co.uk
Website: www.super-food.co.uk

Index